Life is Eximius Ordo

Nigel Shaun Downing

Life is Eximius Ordo

To Jane,

Stars made from Stardust,

[signature]

Olympia Publishers
London

www.olympiapublishers.com
OLYMPIA PAPERBACK EDITION

A CIP catalogue record for this title is
available from the British Library.

ISBN: 978-1-84897-595-8

(Olympia Publishers is part of Ashwell Publishing Ltd)

This is a work of fiction.
Names, characters, places and incidents originate from the writer's
imagination. Any resemblance to actual persons, living or dead, is purely
coincidental.

First published *in 2016*

Olympia Publishers
60 Cannon Street
London
EC4N 6NP

Printed in Great Britain

For my parents - for their never ending patience and understanding.

Acknowledgements

Thanks to Helen Boutle and Hayley Youell at Creative Recovery. Without you both, this would not have been possible. Also to Alan Brookes and Colin Speakman – you both know why.

This collection of poems were written in various stages of my illness, that being Bipolar Affective Disorder.

They were created in my attempt to understand my life and illness as well as the World around me through those eyes.

Some were written when I was slightly manic, or more so, yet others when I was suicidal, and some where I was somewhere in the middle.

I hope you enjoy my journey, although it's been a bumpy ride!

CONTENTS

NEED I SAY ANYMORE?... 15

GLANCE.. 17

EVERYWHERE 18

I DRINK TO 19

THINKING 20

ALCOHOL... 21

FUNFAIR IN THE SKY 22

THESE DAYS... 23

THE ORB-SERVATORY.. 24

THE MIRROR 25

MERCURY RAIN 26

FIRESIDE 27

MAN IN THE MOON 28

I THINK WITH CLARITY 29

BLUE 31

SO I'D SAY. 32

BLANK PAGE.. 33

PAINTING PICTURES 34

YOU CLOTHED AND BATHED ME.............................. 35

ROCKETS... 36

SUNBEAMS ON MY FACE.. 37

BLACK FOG 38

EBB AND FLOW 39

BIRDS 40

SKIN 41

ON THOUGHT 42

PAIN 43

GHOST SOLDIER 44

LIGHTS OUT 45

WALKING INTO THE SUN 47

THIS BREEZE 48

PENCIL ME IN 49

WHEN A TEAR.. 50

YOUR EYES ARE OPEN 52

BACK IN THE SWIM... 53

SELFLESSNESS 55

AS TO SLEEP.. 56

BURNING BRIDGES... 57

F.Y.I.O. 58

FALLEN... 60

FOUR O'CLOCK 61

THE TEMPEST 62

HARD 63

IS IT BECAUSE?.. 65

SLEEP 67

TEACH ME HOW 69

THE DARKNESS 71

NEEDLES 72

DOCUMENT ONE 73

EERIE 75

SECRET THUNDER.. 76

THE DOOR... 77

THE FAT CONTROLLER 79

THE MAGIC SWITCHES 80

THE TRAIN 81

THE UGLY SPECTRE 82

WEAR THE CROWN (PART 1) 84

WEAR THE CROWN (PART 2) 86

WHO? 88

NEED I SAY ANYMORE?

On the last night, when you said that you were leaving,
We gave each other promises we longed to believe in.
Said if we were given down the book of time,
We'd be laid out in the stars,
Well, we never fought to reason
With what we thought was ours.
I'd thought we'd play it out to the very end,
Guess I'll go it on my own,
You know I'll always be your friend,
But just before you go, tell me now:
How could I ever prove? I've nothing more to lose.
So cut it any which way you choose,
I'll be running, running for the rest of my life,
Sleeping with my back on the edge of a knife,
'cause I could never write you down,
I could never paint you up,
You were everything within my soul:
So, need I say anymore?
What's right? While you were still breathing,
We made each other promises, wrong to be leaving,
If it was given in these hands of mine,
I'd pray out to the stars,
Well who taught us there's a reason,
For this love of ours,
I know we played it out to the very end,

You're leaving me now, my only friend.
Now, as I see you go,
I could never choose to cut you loose,
But any which way, I'll have to prove
I'll be running, running for the rest of my life,
Sleeping 'til you turn back on the light,
'cause should I ever write you down,
I could never pick you up,
You were within, in everything-my soul:
So need I say anymore?
You lost the fight and I saw you leaving,
Brave belongs the Promised Land you now live in,
We were given by The Hand, between the lines,
You ray out from the stars,
I'll see you in all the seasons,
Through all this love of ours,
I'd hoped we'd make it through the fairy-tale,
So thank Him for the loan,
We'll always be together,
You've always held my soul,
So how could I ever lose? I'll cut a river to prove,
I'll be running, running for the rest of my life,
Sleeping 'til we're together in the Light,
'cause should you ever ride on down:
You'd forever pick me up...
I'm living, but not within,
For my everything, my soul-

Need I say anymore?

GLANCE

Most people think they can read me,
Like they're looking at a book.
Flick across the pages:
Excuse me-take another look.
Yeah, check out the cover,
Or a glance at the contents page,
But should you miss the story-line,
You've lost the centre stage.
For I am not a quick flick,
Second look or a casual glance:
I'm a fightin' soul livin' in a world,
Where we have but just one chance,
So if you can only read so deep,
As no further than a glance and not a stare;
I guess I'd rather leave you,
Where a glance is not a care.

EVERYWHERE

When I'm watchin' TV I sit and stare,
I change the channel, but you're still there,
Well, the radio's been playin' on all day,
But you were the tune and the words they say.

So I walk alone on a lonely street,
But I still hear you in the fall of my feet.
Then I see a stranger so unaware,
He doesn't know that you're still there,
As I pass, I give a smile quite anew,
After all, My Love

He never knew you.

I DRINK TO . . .

I drink to remember,
I drink to forget,
And though the evening is nearly over,
My life's not over yet.
I drink when I am lonely,
Find my partner in the night:
Such good friends, yet enemies,
In a never ending fight.
From a waltz to a trance,
We dance 'til we drop,
A seductive induction,
Without a mental full-stop.
A roller-coaster ride from hell!
Without the ticket of submission,
A scream so loud it's from all sides!
The price of your admission.
But for all your caress without a cause,
Like a whore off on the run,
I'd rather you left me where I was found:
And my life had just begun.
I think if I remember,
Times I'd rather forget-
Years gone by in a relationship:

And I'm surrounded… by regret.

THINKING

NEED TO STOP DRINKING,

NEED TO START THINKING,

NEED TO FIND A FUTURE,

WITH A ROSY ALLURE.

NEED TO FIND ANSWERS,

TO CURE MY OWN CANCERS-

OR I'LL BE DEAD.

FOR SURE.

ALCOHOL

Good-bye old friend,
You were never there;
You never stopped to say you care.
So it's off with the old,
And in with the new,
Sorry my stranger,
But I never knew you.
For all the conversation,
The fun and the games,
You never once gave me,
Where you took the blame.
I'll say this once,
Though I know it's not nice:
You are the one that let me pay-
Oh but such a heavy price!
Yes you were fun, polite, and oh so right,
But it's not a good game to stand here and fight.
So farewell, ahoy - to friendships new,
Sorry my friend,

I never knew you.

FUNFAIR IN THE SKY

You move so fast like nothing won't last:
Except the lies you spin.
Keep moving around like your feet won't touch the ground:
But you don't know where they've 'bin.
You live for your lovers, chasin' the crazy colours,
They can't see you're living a lie.
You give your love on a merry-go-round,
On a funfair in the sky.
The victims behind show the number of times,
That you've played out your game.
You always aim to win don't you know it's a sin,
To leave them with all your blame?
You don't know how to feel just give them a show-reel,
From the silver screen -
An actor, from the start, just playing a part,
In a movie scene,
That's why you give your love on a merry-go-round,
On a funfair in the sky.
You live for your lovers, to chase the crazy colours,
But they are the ones that die.
For who pays the cost when the love in you is lost,
And their lives' left torn apart,
Do they all find at the back of their mind:

They were a victim from the start?

THESE DAYS

These days I walk alone in the dark,
With nowhere to call home.
Shadows of my past surround me
They chill me for their tone.
I look around at chasing shadows,
The past grinding at my bones.
Set ahead is a narrow road,
Deep in front of a sea,
A time and a land I need to find,
The somewhere they call "me".
Though I laugh when I am scorned,
I'll carry on though weary and worn.
For when I take a look deep inside,
Though the land I seek is far from me,
I see an ocean wide:
That which lives within one's self,
The one that they call pride.
And however my fate is chiselled out,
I know it from that past:
I'm using my own compass,
And that compass is my mast,
So come forth the storm,
Come forth the strife,
You cannot wreck me,
For I have a life.

THE ORB-SERVATORY

Sitting in a café by a doorway to the street,
Lookin' at all the faces, but they're starin' at their feet,
Just twistin' and a turnin' tryin' to find a place,
A pantomime on a show in time just keepin' up the pace.
Livin' in a rat-race, everybody takin' a part-
No time to be learnin',
A thief stole you from the start.
Livin' in a rat-race, fightin' for a space,
No time to stop they pass you by,
Well how are you now I'm doin' fine?
Standing in a hall-way, waiting out my turn,
Listening to fat-cats, braggin' 'bout what they earn,
Twisted stomach burning, watched smiling he signed the bill,
You run the ride, please mind aside:
You people make me ill.
Look into your wallets, for what you can't find in your hearts,
Nothing for a nation, that money tore apart,
Just jestin' at what you invest in, aimed only at one goal,
A fuel in a duel, playing the fool,

You burned away your soul.

THE MIRROR

When I look into the mirror,
Every now and then,
Just before I shiver:
I take a look again.
I see a face there right beside me,
Where she used to be,
A window to a world,
Where I used to see.
And I'm taken back by it all,
Before the past made these days have walls.
You and I under silver blues,
Wondering wild through crimson hues,
How on earth could we ever lose?
In a second before I fall,
I look back at the mirror on the wall.
If I look into the window,
For the why and when,
All I'd see in the corners is that place again:
A place there to remind me,
Of how I used to see,
A vision of a world,
Where I'd rather be.

MERCURY RAIN

A patter of rain on my window pane,
Kickin' up feelings pumpin' through my veins,
Just caught up with being framed in time,
Chasing paranoia around in my mind,
Starin' at faces to the sound of a beat,
So colour me a rainbow and I'll show you my streets.
A buzz in my head says I'm better off dead -
But I'm writing books none of you have read,
Profanity and vanity are two of your needs,
The devil and his sanctuary are sowing your seeds.
The clatter of chains in a mercury rain,
Leaning up at ceilings thumping with my pain,
Just bought up with blame for a time,
Facing Pandora in sound now I'm blind.
Uncovering traces I feel found at my feet,
Go cover me in stains though I'll hold in the heat.
You're chasin' my veins just to drive me insane,
Sealin' out ya meaning losing's not my game,
Just fought up to your shame for a time,
Chaste to ignore what you've found now I'm fine.
I'm glistening, still listening, from under your feet,
Gone over your whole show-
Just dust on your streets.

FIRESIDE

Waiting by the fireside,
To ride away with my dreams tonight,
So far away from the shadows of my life.
It's the only way I know,
To get to where I want to go.
Oh no, why do I only live and breathe,
To chase after dreams to take me away,
Wakin' every morning to live out the same day?
Take me as I am but take me now:
I know I ain't no preacher but I know I need a prayer,
I'll give you all my hands could ever hold and thank you for ever
more,
'till the rivers run dry from the corner of my eyes,
I need to feel my dreams:
That's where she lives so it seems.
So when I'm fallin' through the flames tonight,
I see her in my dreams on the other side,
And try what I may in the fall of night,
She's the only one I know,
Who took me where I want to go,
Now I only live to breathe,
Forever after riding dreams,
That break me every day,
Wakin' every morning,

Living out the same way.

MAN IN THE MOON

Man in the moon say I a crazy guy,
She shine down on me and I cannot lie,
For she carries me along her tides,
The Goddess above, allows me to ride.
Her creator shines through, over to this Earth,
And allows me to fight for all we are worth:
They put me here to carry us through,
Shackled to the Word, whatever we do.
Through the darkest of days,
Out of the dim bright of night,
They voyage me along the times,
To bring you to the Light:
A torch in the day,
And a sword in the night,
Here to carry over,
What we know to be right.
Some say we tick, some say we tock,
Between the sun and the moon,
And your concept of clock–
We are the ones who say when we stop.

I THINK WITH CLARITY

I think with clarity, speed and grace, that's why there's a smile
upon my face,
You think I'm high but I don't know why, my speech is not
pressured but equally measured,
To match my mood so I find it rude,
And though you judge I hold no grudge,
For you were before me so I guess you can call me,
But it's not your place to end my race for time and space within
my kind,
Is only relative to the speed I find.
I'll be kind I'm sure while you try a cure,
You cannot hold me and though you scold me:
I ain't perplexed though you're leaving me vexed,
So may I be so bold as to have it told,
I am just a happy guy and your stories getting old.
But my story could be sent with endless unrelent,
Ashamed of what you meant with all your malicious intent,
For you've got the rant and you've got the rave,
But I ain't the one taking the boring life,
Into an early grave.
So I'll set the stage while you write and turn the page, then I'll run
another mile,
While you try to remove my smile.
For all your writings and your books it only took me the time to look,
At all the rats in your race,
And if I'm honest I don't like the pace,

So guess I'll hold it steady while your psychiatric pen is ready,
'cos I'll just lean upon this sword if you chain me to your ward,
And what I'd be saying if this was it,
Is you doctors are full of sh*t!
So leave me alone don't try to bring me down from this simple
basic philosophy I've found:
If we're only here once I'll take it at my measure,
You were not born with any single right,
To deny me of my pleasure,
and if life is simple, hard and fast,
Easy to waste and not meant to last-
Keep your next prescription Mr Physician!
Shall I put an end to your war or are you the one unable to judge,
And am I coming back for more?
For you are the one who will go insane,
Of that I am definitely sure!
You cannot cure me of happiness for loving life so pure,
For being successful at life itself whatever you put in the way,
So come what may try me today,
Guilty on count of crimes,
And thinking far ahead of you and living in your times,
YOU JUST HAVEN'T GOT A CLUE SO NOW IT'S UP TO YOU:
I think with clarity, speed and grace,

That's why there's a smile
Upon my face.

BLUE

When you are down and feeling blue,
Think of us looking back at you,
For an ocean, however deep or wide,
Cannot hide the emotion,
We give you from inside.
You may think that no-one can hear you,
You may think that no-one cares:
But close your eyes and feel us,
And we will be right there,
When you are lost we'll be your guide,
And catch you when you fall.
Just remember us in times of trouble-
We'll be there before you call.
Some say that we are angels,
But we are just your friends:
With the map of life between us,
To take us to the ends.

SO I'D SAY. . .

So I'd say to Lloyd Webber we all think we're very clever,
But Monet and Freud honed my senses to never never,
Warmed my hearts fire with their aims,
So I started falling apart in my dreams.
And I'm finding the point of undecided decision:
Where the ra ra at the seat of this ranting,
Results from a derision,
See if you take confused as the final answer,
You'd have to state your relativity,
To surf along the central,
Hyper dimensional testing terrestrial,
If? How? Why? When?
Then it hurts!
So I plane off my pain the Law Lords way,
To cut me back to my roots.
And with my boots intact they ride this raft,
Amongst with the waters and up with the air,
Riding the line between the truth of my imagination,
Almost at the point of the tip of my mind,
Crackin' its whip at the final destination.
So I'd say to Lloyd Webber we all think we're very clever,
But Monet and Freud honed my senses to never never.

BLANK PAGE

Blank page takes centre stage,
Pen pushing through the past,
Your mind is blank:
No words to write,
But the ink seems to land so fast.
No purpose other than incarceration,
To run out its own duration,
When words are found,
Yet unwritten then lost,
Emotions unbound,
To run in their sound,
Titled "Unwritten" they pay the cost.
Yet now all I find,
At the back of my mind:
Tis I that is truly lost!

PAINTING PICTURES

If words are painting pictures,
From somewhere deep inside,
And to write is to unfold the canvas within,
Painting out from where we hide:
I fathom that I scare myself,
On the colours that I ride.
The mood I find within myself,
Would therefore truly depend,
On where I leave my brushstrokes,
And where I draw the ends.
For wherever I hang is wherever I look,
Whatever I write is all that it took.
Yet but the limit of your vision,
Would be somewhere deep within,
Just pockets and the odd corner,
Where I have let you in.

YOU CLOTHED AND BATHED ME

You clothed and bathed me when I was young,
You held my life when it had just begun,
You nurtured me and watched me grow,
You gave me thoughts and all I know.
You hold me in my troubles,
And bridge me in my cares,
You gave me love unconditionally,
Bestowed to me your wares-
You will never be not needed,
Though you may be far away,
And I am within a part of you,
Every second of the day,
So although I may sometimes miss,
A thank-you or a smile,
You never let go of my hands,

You walk my every mile.

ROCKETS

We are built from the tree of life, and we are from the tree of life,
So enough of this toil, enough of this strife,
It's crystal clear:
We are but the breeze on the leaves.
Yet but this daily grind I find,
Is bringing me to my knees:
We're all grown from the soil, but it makes my blood boil-
"Send rockets to outer space,
To further the human race".
Yet here, the toil and the till, is making us ill,
Total compassion is without a trace.
It's down in this land, that God needs a hand:
The taste of our own bitter pill.
Famine and wars with unjustified cause-
The collective of the whole human mill.
In pockets we find, there's only one of a kind-
The collective unconscious holds only one face,
Where money has no value,
And disappears without a trace,
So go now,
Send your rockets into space.

SUNBEAMS ON MY FACE

What is this upon my face that caresses me with warm embrace?
So truly delightful inciting such glee,
With a strange glow as if just for me!
To show in my smile and give lift to my walk,
And as I talk a strange air of grace.
Can life's treasures be bought from such simple pleasures?
If not what would be the measure to ensue?
I'm certain if there were no more,
Then I would be cold of heart and mood,
But I see it there for sure:
So pure in its innocent honesty,
Or maybe it's just me.
But as sure as it goes not only I know,
Beyond a shadow and a trace,
Nothing can beat as I walk down the street–

Those sunbeams on my face!

BLACK FOG

Black fog black fog leave me alone,
Why do you always find me,
When I am on my own?
Black fog black fog in the middle of the day,
Black fog you fill me with dismay.
Why cannot you be the light,
And fill me instead with delight?
Why do you have to fill me with the darkness,
And run distress?
And turn darkness into weep,
From something into nothing-
A twisting oh so deep.
Black fog black fog:
Where no-one else is there,
Black fog black fog:
Where no-one else can care.
Black fog black fog,
Why do you stand there and stare?
Black fog black fog,
Why is it you do not care?

EBB AND FLOW

Where does it go, this ebb and flow?
As intricate as a spiders' web:
'cept one minute you're alive, and the next second-you're dead.
In one minute you're gone, from singing a song,
One heart beat stood on two feet,
Then back to a crawl and a stall,
And another tick, and you love it all:
Then back to lamenting, presenting the resenting,
Of the day you were born,
Yet wishing you had another day just to go out and play.
And so the ebb and flow.
How I wish it would go -
I'm tired and need to go to bed,
For this aching head has the beats of the streets,
In all, in awe:
At the fitting of my feet–

And I'm not beat!

BIRDS

When I watch the birds they slow down time,
And I disappear to a world that's mine,
So I often stop, look and listen-
And wonder why?
For they go about their business without a second care or thought,
Living in their own carefree micro world,
Wherein nothing we were taught,
And I'm caught in the wonder of their majesty,
A creation sent surely to please.
Though I slow down the time and make the moment mine,
It's the Creator who provides for their needs.
And with a soar and a dive they bring me alive,
And bring my soul up closer to the sun-
So I hover in their moment,
Before reality has won.
So when you look at the birds as they pass you by-
Stop look and listen,
And wonder why?

SKIN

It's a tragedy this bipolarity,
Wish I could peel it off like old skin.
Then underneath of course, without a lack of remorse,
I'd find a starting place from where to begin.
But as it is now I have to find somehow,
Where the wild horses are only ridden in leisure,
And the pleasure of a kind, that tears and rips at my mind,
Is solely given for me to treasure-
Not to run and trash, make me behave so unabashed,
Like a stallion set on the loose.
For when temperaments reigned back in,
The beginning is back to begin.
Regrets a plenty for all those abused,
Yes a manic mind is one of a kind,
But it's one I'd rather lose!
But when I look at my skin, it looks good from within,
And I've only got one thing to prove-

I've only myself to remove.

ON THOUGHT

What is this: that I sit here and think with?
And who is this: that I think here and drink with?
What is me that is truly profound?
Yet sits in silence: but speaks with no sound.
And as I hear, alone, to whom is it I listen?
For if self is found in sound,
Then the sound must be my soul?
And if my soul can hear itself,
Have I found my goal?

PAIN

Pain – let's talk about pain.
It has a thought,
That leads to a vein.
A vein so central,
It becomes hyper-mental,
Like standing out cold in the rain.
It's cold and hard,
And constantly beating-
Like the heart inside,
Has no unfold for its treating.
Nothing to show,
Nowhere to go,
Nothing for the standing,
No tears to run,
Nothing to face,
Nothing for a beating.
No-one has won,
Nothing has passed,
It's the unfortunate ones who walk by,

With nothing in them to last.

GHOST SOLDIER

As my spirit flies I can tell no more lies:
See I'm acted upon and then sent, down the vein of time itself.
Living here amongst others-
All my sisters and my brothers.
See I see time as nothing but divine, to put the spaces making gaps,
Perhaps you do not understand the clock.
But I need nothing for a sword, or my hands upon a Glock,
My nine millimetre lives on both hands,
My spirit lives in your theatre, as I walk upon your lands.
See spirit for all seven colours, surrounded on my head,
Curse thyself among me,
Where enemy see out in red.
The dread you must find at the back of your mind,
Is I am white while you are dead.
See my spirit now, when I give you grace!
My Lord and Master runs this place!
So go now run find where you begun,
But carry me not to your wars,
For we are here because of Him,

And I just play out his cause.

LIGHTS OUT

Who turned the lights out? Who made it all scream and shout?
Who made it all collide,
From every angle deep inside?
Who gave it all, all this thrust into no-one that man can trust?
Who turned the white into total black?
Who put my own colours into one attack?
Who took my truth and turned them into lies?
Who gave me my white and turned them through that black?
Who counted me yet forgot me in the mount,
As I fly in darkness waiting for the count?
To surmount this dark stallion I do not wish to ride!
It's reign within a lack of hope:
And to choke on its black smoke,
Living as I breathe trying to retrieve,
A will somewhere in a want-a magic wand I must weave:
For somewhere near on choke.
For it is surely one dark ghost that forever I would not wake:
Nor would I wish to give it life, never-for my sake,
To ride these horses must be a sin, six-fold of them to one of me,
With many hooves and their clatter and din!
Take me away as fast as they arrived, their energy from black-
Time out now I have seen them, it's my life that's under attack.
At last-they're contrived from my own mind,
see it now as I see it clear:

I have one horse near!
My horse is white and through the darkness of this night,
As a knight I have rode her along.
Through the fear I rein her near,

And she has won all along.

WALKING INTO THE SUN

Walking into the sun often sounds like oh so much fun:
For when you're down and beat,
And off your feet,
It just seems to all make sense, in all its recompense.
A repose to a suppose that all will be fine.
It's in the sublime just for a chance to change,
And though it now seems strange,
It's a change I must take-but tentatively and not negative.
For this must surely be better,
Than walking into the sun.

THIS BREEZE

On this breeze if you please:
The ghost scent of nature has old soul,
Sent for those who listen for the Tryst:
And glisten and listen for its goal.
Toying with branches but never taking chances:
The long run to keep up the whole,
Alive in its drive to keep us alive:
A trusted story already sold.
Keep wing in sky and cloud adrift,
Fast fancy past, spent out for the thrift-
Feel magic on the face if you slow down the pace.
The sweet magic touching on skin:
When you realise when you open your eyes -
The air is where we begin.
True, close and free, free of our sin,

Yet softly, gently, it touches our skin.

PENCIL ME IN

Please, Creator, pencil me in.
Put me in today, but free from sin:
Put me in forever, and then for a day,
Put me in always, come what may.
For always in the strife and always in the cleave,
For always in the want and always in the need.
Bring me to you but pencil me in:
Send me forth free from sin,
Pencil me in as one with you,
Pencil me in and make me true.
Pencil me in as high as the sky,
Lead me to the truth and away from the lies.
Pencil me in for one more day,
Pencil me in from that in which may lead us astray.
Pencil me in from sin as it is taught,
Pencil me in from that in which I can be bought,
Pencil me in, if only for one day-

Pencil me in, come what may.

WHEN A TEAR

When a tear, feels oh so near:
Just look up to the sky.
When pain envelopes and you cannot cope:
Leave out the question as to why.
For a reprieve if you believe, will come back to you,
When it feels oh so real in that envelope of terror, that you find
when you're on your own:
Don't try to run faster and further away:
See the lies you tell yourself,
The fear left to grow and build,
For sake of lack of coping, or so it seems and feels,
No hope is not the answer:
For today the dread must be read,
Grasped, gripped and whipped:
Into shape from an untrustworthy form,
Like a penny cast adrift for a wish,
To the water and far out to sea-set it free.
The lies seen against the shimmering,
Of hope and a glint of glee:
Dark cloak removed and sent out adrift,
Despair named as the demon evil at its craft:
So plain now for all to see.
So when the darkness descends, do not fear,
Just look up to the sky...
hold it near,
For one glimmer of light,

And the answer as to why.

YOUR EYES ARE OPEN

Your eyes are open but they cannot see.
Your heart is open but it casts no glee.
All is blank and undesired:
Your mind is weak and you're getting tired.
Your feet land heavy but they know no wait,
The sword you carry is for one last fight.
So in the dark you stab and in the dark you parry:
Murder of a kind to which you must marry.
Carry not a chink in your armour:
But fight for a chink of pure light,
For today and tomorrow unto it you must follow,
And carry on 'till you know I am right.
The strife and the strafe is only for the brave,
Faint of heart need not apply,
For none of us question ourselves,

Or ever wonder, why?

BACK IN THE SWIM

It's nice to be back in the swim!
From the deep,
To the surface.
And then to the shore: the hunger and its lasting,
That makes you reach out for more,
Dead to the was but still dying,
Sinking fast,
Then current lost,
And depth for past, destiny-the floor.
Yes destiny the bottom,
Ocean to swallow, and leave you forgotten.
But in the hearts last dying ember, of one last fire:
It's a glimmer of hope and trust that halts,
Then lifts us higher.
An institution of evolution:
Pain intact,
But nestling in comfort of emotive thought.
So then we lift,
To the surface then drift...
In waves lost but in a retort:
A thin sliver of a swimmer,
And just a shade too close to a trance -
An un-denied trance
Glancing then fast:
But dancing.
Without doubt, a glimmer in a sea,

53

A matter, alive in this universe-
A conscious self of me!
So swim I can,
And swim I will.
Out of this ocean and onto the beach
Within my matter, un-denied,
I have swum so fast.
And found the need to hide:
Yet I am not an empty shell,
Lying at the bottom of the sea:
I can see the shore, where I can be once more-

Back to the being they call me.

SELFLESSNESS

If you look into the shadows,
You will find me there.
I've no time to be in the lime-light,
For that I do not care-
See, I choose to do my moving,
Improving all I may,
In just small steps and pieces,
Gathered in the day.
Take shells of people and make them whole,
A better self-
The only goal.
To weave and wind,
By being kind,
And laughing all along,
An ear to bend,
And a shoulder to lend,
In quiet moments when things go wrong.
The song I sing is a whistle in my mind,
For quietness is in the victory,
Lives out in the proof I find,
When easy effort is the truth-

Yes the product of being kind.

AS TO SLEEP

Let autumn be the favourite season,
Senescence all around,
The silent beauty of nature's sleep,
Above and below the ground.
'till warmer climes lay upon them,
They look as if to wither and die:
But you and I know their secret,
Still showing beauty as they lie.
Who is to say when nature,
Is showing herself at best-
But is it found in autumn,
When nature takes a rest?

BURNING BRIDGES

I've done with all this walking:-
The endless chattering,
And all its talking.
It's time to stop, turn, and move on.
The prolonged-ness of the etching at my brow-
An end to this to find somehow.
I've lost the way as it feeds,
Where my mind wanders as it weaves.
I've lost the right path somehow,
With a torturous kind of attention,
To these weaving leaves at my feet-
I make no mention-
Of my past so ugly and so loud,
And as the needles of life dig deep into me,
The crossroad ahead I scarcely see,
Then I'm stood so proud...
So with one more step,
And a shake of my old boots-
I'll follow the map as found,
Back to the roots at my feet,
It's straight ahead now-

No time for defeat.

F.Y.I.O.

My father would do anything,
He wears no crown, but he is king!
Ask him to walk a mile,
And he would walk another inch,
To ask him out loud for the helping hand,
He'd do so without a flinch.
He's picked me up when I've been down,
He's not laughed at me,
When I've been a clown.
He's carried my weight when I could not fight,
And cushioned the blow,
When I wasn't right.
He'd take on my assailants,
And all my mental ailments,
And believes in me when I am right.
He points me towards the truth,
When neither he nor I can smatter a proof,
But surely and surly,
He puts in the pin,
My father is always certain,
Of when my battle will win.
He knows my life and when it will hurt,
The evil-minded women,
Who treated me like dirt…
He knows my silent wounds,
And how they have cocooned me so deep,

He knows how the years have cut into my tears,
And why I am steel to a weep.
A mettle to fight in life's seasons,
A hardened caution to this my world,
A man to give me reasons,
And strength he holds in quiet times,
Dusts off small pieces to be mine.
My father would do anything,
But commit no crime,
Or perform any sin.
Yet my father is just my dad,
And for that fact,

I am surely glad.

FALLEN

She's narcotic, she needs to stop it,
Don't she know I need see sense?
It's in her innocence as she smiles:
Sends me skyward for miles.
I'd walk the proverbial distance just to catch the glint in her eye,
Where I die and am reborn again:
A thousand times in a second.
She does not know her recompense,
Or that I am a man already reckoned,
To meet another who has fallen, from much the same old place,
Where the history of man himself, is in one smile on her face.
See angels know as they go, they must be carefree,
And act not unlike mere mortals:
But that's not her and me.
I know to her as she knows it can be, that two together can truly,
Be footloose and fancy-free,
It may be forbidden for us, as we are from the skies:
But glints in eyes can cut so deep,
There's no room for any lies.
Truth is told but seldom seen,
Felt deep in the heart on one white gleam,
So see her now and see her beam,
Powerless in thought that we know what drives us:
The lesson that He taught...

That He is behind us

FOUR O'CLOCK

TICK-TOCK IT'S FOUR O'CLOCK,
WHILE EVERYONE'S SNORING,
I'M FINDING IT BORING,
STARING AT THE CEILING,
LOOKING FOR A MEANING.
WIDE-EYED AND WIDE AWAKE,
MAKE NO MISTAKE,
NO REST FOUND IN THIS HUM-DRUM SOUND,
NO DREAMS TO GIVE AND NO DREAMS TO TAKE,
FOR SAKE OF SANITY GIVE ME A BREAK,
FOR I TRULY TAKE THIS ALL THE TIME-
GIVE IT BACK THIS MIND IS MINE,
TRULY RAMBLING AWAY IN A BUBBLE,
BUT GIVE IT BACK ALTHOUGH IT'S TROUBLE,
PEACE OF MIND IS ALL I ASK,
WHY SHOULD IT BE SUCH A HEAVY TASK?
IS IT TOO MUCH TO ASK,
FOR PEACE OF A KIND?
AS THERE'S NO SPACE LEFT,
IN MY CROWDED MIND.

THE TEMPEST

The tempest has her growl around me,
But soft heart beats inside:
The toying thoughts that lay cast around are free,
Warm hearts fire cast abound in me.
Her tears they rain on down,
And sting upon my face:
Embraced am I as she plays at leisure,
Humbled am I to share her pleasure.
Weather she is and whether she isn't-
I'm grateful to her for wonderful present,
For present am I in her at her free will:
And thanking her for my presence,
For life she has brought,
For wind and rain I cannot blame,

Her gift to me she has taught.

HARD

It's hard to describe what I feel inside,
When mind moves faster than a wander.
When to plunder the deep dark depths,
Will tell time on days a plenty,
When the speed of light feels nothing but right,
And running right off the meter:
Where my feet matches my mind,
And both travel many miles:
Where smiles are all I have-
And given out a plenty.
But many frowns I see in return,
Yet but the burn of love,
And the happiness,
Is bursting from inside,
And my heart has no-where to go,
Or a single wish to hide-
No need to sleep or the want to weep,
For the ones around me,
Who just do not understand:
They see before them a jibber-jabber wreck,
Strange, eccentric, and to avoid,
And no reason to it all,
Just someone to avoid.
Where a chance and fast encounter with me,

Always leaves them annoyed,
Where reality has been left behind,
With no reminder or recall.
But happy now as happy is-

This bipolar mania,
Is a total jizz.

IS IT BECAUSE?

Is it because I stole a pencil from school?
Was it then, that you made the rule?
If you are bipolar then stand on my shoulder-
I can carry enough weight for two.
For those without the doors have a get out clause-
They don't really have a clue.
Is it because I don't get along,
With everyone with whom I am found?
Is it because I am far from a saint,
And all that glimmers in me is not gold?
Is it because the Thou has cast me-
A man to learn a lesson?
Or is it because I aim to cast only glee,
And you are but a devil in me?
Is it because my mind can be unclean and untidy,
And the Thou has taken me for an untimely ride?
Is it because I love this Earth,
And all the people and what they are worth?
Are my intentions too good and my heart too true?
And is the devil at work between me and the truth?
For if he's close behind me I need a clue.
Is it because I did not succeed in that all I set sail,
Or that I tried through all the avail?
Is it because I see the ill in others,
Then choose them not to be friends,
When, patience if lasted out,

Would join us in the ends?
Is it because of lack of submitting pure patience
Of others so found denied?
If I run in my mind what would I find-
Except that which is at a total loss?
Look at my cost.
Is it because I try too hard,
To see shining in others and not me?
Or is it because I weigh up too much,
And the answer lies in those who are free?
Then still am I clouded in vision and thought,

In the bipolarity they call me!

SLEEP

If you lay there silent when there's no more proving,
With saint by your soul,
And your Lord to your side:
You truly live,
Where there's no-where to hide.
Naked and pure,
You know for sure,
That it's the silence that makes the sense.
The actions of your truth land you in purity,
At one with the Word in your sanctuary,
So on with this silence and off with this land,
It's off to the slumber,
In one gentle Hand.
The day is over and another to begin:
Another start,
Where the good will win.
It's fair to start in the closing of your eyes:
The good you will do,
Where the devil will despise,
For a heart like yours forever to be true,
To a God like yours,
Is between Him and you,

.

So if you lay there silent

You'll make just appear His Word,
And the conversation between yourselves,
Is private and unheard,
For saints and souls will make you brave:
And lift you up to your sleep,
Where the angels and one true God,
Are there for you to keep.

TEACH ME HOW

Teach me how to kiss again,
For I have been just a fool.
No rule to follow but my own sense,
Where my mind is caught up in a duel.
There was lost and found then I floundered,
And further lost just in the thought:
In touching lips and one tight grip-
And the scorn of one big retort.
When you hide from an adventure,
Instead of thanking for what he sent ya,
Spinning and turning,
With your own stomach churning,
Feeling like you'll turn up the ghoul,
Like kissing back at school-
Pleasant lady in the present,
Yes looking oh so pleasant!
Like there's only one thing left to do-
So teach me how to kiss again,
Upon this pane kissed with the rain,
As I'm fraught with fight to get it right,
Before I stand at night with her again.
Must I endure the pain,
To see her go?
Then I kiss my soul…
And for another day to endure-
Will I be sure the next time we meet,

That our lips touch-and all will be sweet,
Oh teach me now to kiss again!
To tell me now I was a fool,
But kiss me now,
And for that to be, then kiss me,

The fool.

THE DARKNESS

ENTER THE DARK TUNNEL,
ENTER AT YOUR PERIL,
MAKE NO MISTAKE THERE'S NO-ONE TO TAKE,
YOUR'E THERE TO MEET THE DEVIL!
TO TORTURE YOU WILL GO,
NO LIGHT FOR YOU TO KNOW,
JUST DARKNESS DEEP AND TWISTED,
GONE INTO THE MISTS OF TIME,
WHERE ALL GOES SLOW-
AND MOTION CEASES TO A HALT,
AND BOLTS OF LIGHTNING SURROUND YOU,
AND FIRE TO WALK ON THE GROUND-
WHERE THE ONLY SOUND IS YOUR SCREAMING,
AGAINST THE GLEAMING SCYTHE OF DEATH!
WHERE DEMONS AND THEIR PITCH-FORKS,
ARE THERE TO TAKE YOUR BREATH,
BUT DO NOT FLUSTER YOU WILL BE SOUND-
MUSTER YOURSELF YOU WILL BE FOUND,
SOLDIER ON TO THE SCYTHE AND FORKS,
THERE YOU WILL FIND THAT THEY CANNOT WALK,
CARRY ON OVER, UP, THROUGH AND ABOVE,
SOMEWHERE THERE YOU WILL FIND THE DOVE,
FOLLOW HER 'TIL YOU SEE THE LIGHT,
AND BE TRULY GRATEFUL,
YOU GAVE IT ONE LAST FIGHT.

NEEDLES

Give me my needle!
'cause I am feelin' feeble.
I need its injection,
Just for my own protection.
Under its influence,
The feeling is profound:
To just be lost,
In its sights and sound,
Just enough to make its kill,
To bring me back,
From feeling ill.
The rush of blood,
That feels so good,
Cannot be so wrong!
Oh, just play it to me one more time,
I live to feel its song,
Just one more trip,
Let me feel free,
I love the rush,
Of memory.
And when the bass is in your face,
And sorrow lost,
Without a trace-
I'm not trying to wreck it all,
But put the needle to the record,
Just once more.

DOCUMENT ONE

In the stillness of night,
When darkness has come,
I think to myself-
From where have I begun,
Such tiny pieces,
But how far they unravel,
The distance inside-
How far must I travel?
In fathoms the depths,
At the back of my mind,
Strive for the truth,
Or something of its kind.
I'm blessed with bliss,
Of that I am sure,
And full of love,
That can only be pure.
Answers I ask,
In the task to be told,
Not subtle or succinct,
But so loud and so bold.
For this journey I make,
Each and every day,
Searching for answers,
Come what may.
With tools to sharpen
In my mind,

More questions for the answers,
Is all I find.
From stars to the moon,
From there and back,
Matter from them both,
I do not lack.
With water and fire,
I have been mettled,
Questions in my mind,
Leave me unsettled.
So swim this river,
Wide, deep, and long,
I'd love to know,
Where I belong?
So surely as long,
As my minds net is cast,
It's in my nature-
These questions to ask.

So who am I?
And who would I be?
If I was nothing,
Who would be me?

EERIE

The eerie glow,
Of what I don't know,
A thousand questions in a second.
No-one to tell,
Of your private hell,
No distance closing in the beckon.
Some obtuse-
And some acute,
Questions to the starry sky,
A million more, than every star,

But no answer for the why?

SECRET THUNDER

Deep thunder rolling around in my mind,
Anger with its thrust and no aim,
So I'm waiting for the magic,
Or something of its kind,
For calmness and serenity to become realigned,
Where love and peace are the same.
I wonder, calling to my inner self,
Why I allow others,
To make my life lame.
At times it's so tragic,
'til I've made up my mind,
It's for the others,
To take up the blame.
Put them under, far and away,
Let the anger cease, bring it to its knees,
If not forever-

Then just for today.

THE DOOR

Is it any business of yours,
This mess I find myself in?
Is there anything you can do for me,
Or is my story wearing thin?
Could you do me just one favour,
And then never no more-
When you leave me behind,
Can you close the door?
It's not much I give you,
Just one last small task,
Leave me alone-
It's not much to ask.
See, I've withered you down,
As I have weathered myself:
Lack of understanding within ourselves,
Imperfections of our inner self,
That in which you would destroy me,
In the lack as to know,
I'm tired of the misunderstanding,
So I ask you to go.
I'm sorry for your burdens,
And misconceptions of my words-
It seems that I have worried you
In what you've seen and heard.
See fact is in that which you do not see,
Beyond this fine veneer,

Have you ever looked for me,
When I have been so near?
I will deny that you have tried,
To see me and not the mask,
Died have I a thousand times,
And cried have I the last.
So go now please!
On my knees,
But no beg,
It's in your thoughts not your words,
That made conversation dead.
See I wear bipolar on both shoulders,
Move boulders with my mind,
And your kind cannot carry me,
And as I leave you undefined.
There will be others who will follow you-
But they will stay not long,
And the song I will sing,
Will miss no beat,
And you will long be wrong.
Never no more-
So when you leave me behind,

Can you close the door?

THE FAT CONTROLLER

Where did the flow go?
Why does it ebb so?
There and gone, how?
Get it back, now?
Why does it hurt so?
Why do I feel low?
Does anybody know?
When will the wings begin?
When will my heart sing?
Will changing winds blow?
When will the pain go?
Will I ever know?
Where will the start be?
When will I be free?
When will the dark turn?
When will the embers burn?
Where will the sign be?
Will it just point back at me?
When will the light show?
Will I know where to go?
Why am I lost now?
Will I get back somehow?
Why?
To the fat controller–

Why grant me life bipolar?

THE MAGIC SWITCHES

The magic switches!
They're either off or they're on,
One minute you're weeping-
The next,
Singing a song.
From pounding rain in a storm,
To bright,
Sunny,
And warm.
From laughing with your best friends-
To wishing your life would come to its end.
From fertile land to barren soil-
One minute full strength,
Then weak from the toil.
From the joy of a new-born baby-
To the very spectre of death,
Those magic switches,
Can take your last breath:
Indeed.
Plant a seed,
The seed and that land,
Will give you a hand-
To lift you from the bottom,
And you will need those rain clouds,

To show you what was forgotten.

THE TRAIN

Sitting by the window on a train,
Wondering if my life will ever change its lane,
Wondering if tomorrow,
Will be the same again.
Staring through the vacant window,
Moving away from past,
Shattered dreams or so it seems,
Will the future ever last?
Ticket master gestures me,
To the future as it's beckoned,
Will I see the future through,
And is it already reckoned?
Just one more stop,
And so it starts,
Feet to land,
With one heavy heart.
I'm getting off the train-
The moving on and getting out,
Of this life and all this pain-
Will I ever learn to stop,
Look, and listen to hear myself,
When I walk on through the rain?
Will I learn to ride this life,
When tomorrow is,
Yet another train?

THE UGLY SPECTRE

Ugly spectre you have raised your vicious head,
Dead I feel to the world.
With silence and darkness you have surrounded me,
But it's your truth I find absurd-
You want me to believe I am on my knees,
Never to dance once more-
Your score I know,
Yet I've still to hit the floor.
With dalliance I hold you in contempt,
Attempt me with all your will-
Still I will lie down,
and I will be here still,
You cannot control the magic in me.
Your dark cloak may surround me now,
But somehow I'll wait out your turn,
Put me to the test and do your best,
With your own iron I'll brandish and burn-
For though the end is far from sight,
Don't forget I've seen you before,
Forlorn I may appear just now,
But it's you that waged a war.
Your demons may dwell,
In every room in my mind,
And I may be locked in its cellar,
But stellar am I and lest you forget-
In my house I'm the only dweller,

So open your dark curtains,
Let me see the shine of the moon,
Both of you are waning now,
And I will be home soon.
Learn your lesson and learn it well-
My home is in my heart-
And you are just a hotel,
I will always beat you,

In my own private hell.

WEAR THE CROWN (PART 1)

Oh dear, oh my,
I cannot lie down,
I seem to be wearing,
A mania crown!
Not just alive,
But totally glowing,
All bright and shiny,
Bright coloured thoughts in the flowing!
Unrelenting in its own lamenting,
Light-
So white,
Shiny,
Pure and warm,
To give out its strength,
As I weather the storm.
Fast last chance,
To catch the last thought,
Thinking so fast!
Alas nothing is caught,
A bought up mind,
With no kind of peace,
No gentle persuasion,
Or chance of release.
A ride through hell
Yet one pointed with pleasure,
And no taught to a maxim,

To hold and to measure,
Unguarded,
Unchained,
And surely un-reined,
Oh to catch one moment to treasure!
Obtuse,
Then acute,
To find the square root,
When tight winding lies the path,
So far I have to travel,
When nothing seems to last.
Alas the crown is heavy,
But now I am the king-
Yet now I bow to the mania,

This hideous wretched thing!

WEAR THE CROWN (PART 2)

Slow me down, slow me down:
I don't want to wear this mania crown!
There's a clown in my shoes,
And I cannot choose my mood,
I've spirits for my spirit,
And no longer have need for food,
Calmer times are needed,
Oh how I wish they would!
So tie me down tie me down-
I need to feel the ground,
For my head is full of colours,
And my ears are full of sound.
The constant chatter,
Of this mental clatter,
Feel like its weakening my very bones.
So take me home take me home,
I no longer wish to stray,
I pray now for the ending,
And the start to be today.
So come what may let this be the end-
For this mania crown,
Is no longer my friend,
So let it go now-
Let this be its death,

For I fear now,
I will draw my last breath…
I wish it would go,
As fast as it begun,
To strong calm and silence-

Where I would have won.

WHO?

Who to break the silence?
Who to break the pain?
Who to break the same old thought,
Rolling around again?
Who to touch in moments?
Who to share a tear?
Who to share a tender hug?
Who to just be near?
Who to turn to in the dead of night?
Who to brighten up the day?
Who to hold to steady,
When weakened legs begin to sway?
Who to echo a hearty laugh?
Who to join the wonder?
Who to wander by the side,

'til death do put us under?